Health Provider Sues Client.
WHAT TO DO?

Dental Malpractice.

DOLORES SEFIROT

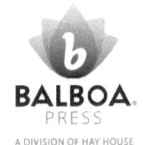

BALBOA.
PRESS

A DIVISION OF HAY HOUSE

Balboa Press books may be ordered through booksellers or by contacting:

Balboa Press
A Division of Hay House
1663 Liberty Drive
Bloomington, IN 47403
www.balboapress.com
1 (877) 407-4847

Print information available on the last page.

ISBN: 978-1-5043-9572-4 (sc)
ISBN: 978-1-5043-9573-1 (e)

Balboa Press rev. date: 01/24/2018

Contents

1

REFUSAL TO THE CALL

As a young girl, I used to dream all the time, in my dreams, the Colorado was running close to our farm. It was named "Rancho Viejo" miles away from the river, but water used to cover this whole area. My Grandpa had started the farm. Later, it became a small town, grandma sold product from the farm and still it was called "Rancho Viejo" In my dreams, I would stride, on the road all covered with stones, and enjoy the sounds the water made. Then it started to speak to me; It sounded like a cat's purring.

Water: "Jump in, my dear. It is cool in here." Sounding "hirrr" like a cat.

I pulled back leaning against a tree trunk, astonished; "What?"

The water repeated; "Do not be afraid, my dear, I'll show you the sea…"

My reaction was to run until I got home, out of breath and scared thinking; "What's that about?"

Next day, my curiosity got the best out of me and again, I dreamed that I went back to the path walking far from the edge. Watching the water fearfully. Suddenly! Water splashed my feet and a giggle came from the water; "You are back!" it purred.

I thought; "This water is too strong. I am not getting in there."

The voice responded to my thoughts; "you will be safe in my medium. Come innn." The voice said dragging its "inn"

I spoke then; "The water churns in the center. I cannot go in there. It's too strong. I am afraid."

And water went on; "You are ready to see the world." It roared and continued smoothly;" It is as big as the ocean. Come inn. I can show you where you were first born."

I got brave and demanded; "Who are you? Why don't you show your face?"

The voice answered with a manly voice; "My name is Eulogio." Showing a hint of deep laughter.

I was startled! Caught my breath and ran home to think: "I will never again go close to the river"

I told myself. I refused the call.

After a while, my dreams started again. And I walked to the river. My steps became faster and secure. Soon I was running to reach the river. I went to the same spot where Eulogio would be waiting. "He will speak to me." I thought and then he surprised me. "Are you enjoying your walk?" and laughed.

I answered, timidly; "Yes."

And he repeated; "Come in the water. I will protect you."

"There are too many quick-sand pools. I know that. I will just walk here, on this side."

Then the dreams changed; it was a different area, and the river was so wide that I could not see the other side of it. In that dream I would take my baby across the river, and Mother was there to help me. I say to her with intense voice; "If baby slips off your arms, let him go."

Mom says enthusiastically; "I can get him back. LOOK!" And she takes a few steps. Therefore; I am in a panic with the realization that I am going to lose them both. I let out a hoarse scream that wakes me up still screaming.

As I got older my dream changed. I wanted to go with Eulogio and cross the river. There was a bridge made of sturdy boards and ropes. I decided to cross the river and fearfully took short steps holding on to the ropes. The water started to splash me and it swirled faster as if trying to pull me in. The struggle became fierce. The ties broke loose and I held on feeling the strength of the water pulling me. I woke up yelling; "NOOO! I am not going."

I looked around and noticed that I was on the

opposite side of the river. "It was a dream only a dream." I told myself. But it really felt shaken. I went to the fields and picked chamomile flowers and made a tea to calm myself.

MY MENTOR; OLD WOMAN

My teacher, "Old Woman" was very old and became my best friend. She was very protective of my security. She taught me to make patch quilts, needle work, played scrabble, talked about school and I told her my secrets. She also decided to give me English classes.

She said, one day. "You and I are going to do business."

I stood up and pulled my dress which had ripped when I climbed off the tree too fast. Old Woman had started to point with her finger towards herself; "I am going to give you classes every day. And you are going to wash my dishes. I HATE to do dishes."

I continued to pull my dress straight and said; "Really? I will ask my Dad's permission."

"NO, it is not necessary. You and I are doing business." She explained pointing at herself and at me with her long bonny finger.

We went at it with a passion. Soon, I was reading the classics on her bookcase. When she saw me reading she asked; "Can you understand this?"

I explained; "I have read them in Spanish already so I can understand most of it."

Old Woman was very pleased with my progress and soon decided that I was old enough to go with her to dances. She became my chaperone too.

There was a CASINO that her husband had started. He was expecting that gambling would be approved in town. He put lots of money and work on it. When the project was not approved, He suffered a stroke, and got around in a golf car. Which I got to use sometimes. What fun!

Then I met a handsome man who came from the

North to enjoy the casino's music. We fell in love and Old Woman approved of him. "Nice Jewish boys make good husbands." She informed me. His family came to meet and we were soon married.

CROSSING THE FIRST THRESHOLD

Actually, I crossed two thresholds. I married into another culture and crossed the border to live within another culture. My teacher; Old Woman had given me a great deal of History, culture and information concerning her family. Her mother died giving birth to Old Woman and she had been brought up by a young slave. When slavery was abolished, both continued close contact until death.

My husband worked for the Southern Pacific Railroad, and soon I met the "gang" They said to me "We are Hillbillies."

I was invited to coffee with the women. And to watch TV; "I Love Lucy" was so much fun. I had the first Thanksgiving Celebration with the whole crew. The gang also included two young brides and I enjoyed their company and instructions on how to shop for my baby.

Being married and a mother brought many changes, of course, after some time moving around, we decided to settle down and moved closer to my family. We had done a great deal of adjusting. We lived together for fourteen years and had three children. Life was good.

Yet, I did not adjust to his ways or his expectations. And I decided to leave. I moved away with the children and got a job to provide for us. I had a job at a school as a teacher's assistant.

Wonderful! I was able to teach English which led to making improvements on my own. I also started college, and made friendships that have lasted for life. I loved to study and to socialize with my friends.

When I finished college, One of the School Administrator, where I worked, asked me if I would be interested in getting a teaching degree. But I was not in a position to go away to study. My children depended on me and I had a house payment.

Then I received an offer: If I worked that year in the summer program, I would be provided with enough pay to cover the money needed to pay off my home. I could start my first session for a teaching degree that year. This was just great for me. I accepted and everything started to fall into place. I received a scholarship from the college teachers which covered rent for three months. The community was very supportive. I was introduced to the staff and felt quite at home at the University Housing.

My children went to the Junior High School there for two years. They were ready to return home when I was offered a scholarship to continue for a Masters degree in teaching. However, I was facing other needs and the children wanted to return home. I turned down the scholarship and a job in the Spanish Department. We returned home.

4

THE ROAD OF TRIALS

I applied for positions and spent much time trying to get an interview from the school that gave me my first break. But there was no position that I could fill. I got jobs that provided for family needs until I could get a permanent position. I also got a job out of the country. But there was nothing permanent for me. What helped was a part-time position at night. I was teaching English as a Second Language for adults.

Then One day, a new Principal was hired in the District. He saw my application, called me and hired me on the spot. "you are just what we need." He stated. I started my job as a teacher which lasted for two years.

The District seemed to have decided that I could not work for them. But I was not informed of any reasons. At the end of the first year, I was not expecting to work the next year. The principal was not informed of the decision, and he provided me with a contract.

That year, all kinds of small things happened. Since the teaching position was my first, I was not aware of problems and some events until one of the old teachers asked me; "What is going on with you? I see that you have all the students who are a problem in the system.

I could not answer. I did not know what "Problematic students" she saw, but she could see it. Another event was clearly "ordered." I had taken over a group of folklore dancers that met after school. The Counselor had been directing it and she asked me to take it over because she had so much work to do.

I had accepted it and we started to practice the dances, having folkloric dresses for the group made, and we were developing long term plans. One of plans was that the group would go on a trip to Europe. We started to take steps. The students were very excited and parents were willing to cooperate as needed. However; plans were not even off the ground when the Counselor came to tell me that she was taking over the group again.

Another event occurred during a Teachers Meeting. The Chair asked a question that did not have a correct answer. He asked me; "What method would you use when a student asks you a question and he/she does not speak English?"

I considered the question and answered; "It would depend on the question."

He insisted; "Would you speak to the student in Spanish?"

I considered it again; "I might speak Spanish if needed."

When we walked out of the session, the Counselor, who spoke Spanish as her native language, commented to me; "You just made a great mistake. It will cost you your job."

I considered the information and looked up the Statutes. There was no law or rule preventing me from speaking Spanish and I wondered; "Wasn't my bilingual status that led to hiring me for that position?"

The next year; there was no Teacher Contract for me. I substituted in the District until I went to see the man who had offered me help to get a Teaching Degree. I asked him what I ought to do so that I could qualify for a teaching position. He leaned back on the desk with his hands joined behind his neck and smiling broadly stated. "You will never work for us. I will see to it."

I did not know what this meant, but I did not ask. Just made a polite gesture with my head and walked away wondering "What was that? it seems personal."

After a few months, I decided to get a Masters in Education with emphasis in Psychology. I understood that the offer to help me get a degree in teaching was meant to keep me away.

But for several years. Administration called me;

"The Loose Cannon." I understood that Administration had something to hide, but I did not know what it was that I "knew". I had enough problems of my own to resolve.

5

THE AUTOMOBILE ACCIDENT

Before starting work at the school I had experienced an automobile accident. During the two years teaching at the District, I had been receiving dental work which started when I had the automobile accident. Four teeth had been broken loose. However; The work had escalated into having a whole bridge which was not working any better than the first "partial" the whole thing had become a serious health problem.

My attention was now on recovering my health. My speech was a problem whether I spoke Spanish or English.

I had been driving through a Country Road;

thinking about the problem with getting a job. I did not want to move away to get work. Just then, I noticed the lights of a car through the fields. I went into high alert! It was clear that the car was coming too fast to stop. It was going to hit me! As it passed the the Stop Sign, I hit the breaks and turned the stirring wheel to the right. The coming car veered to the left. It hit my fender instead of my door. It would have killed me. The impact caused my car to turn in a circle over and over, moving in slow motion. I saw my face in the mirror bounce from the steering wheel until the car stopped on the opposite side of the road.

I wondered about the other cars coming from behind me. I could have a crash again! Every thing was moving in slow motion. I saw the mirror; glass all over my face, shoulder, arm. There was a cut from the top of y nose to the mouth. And a cut on the lower lip. A big gap appeared where four teeth should have been. I looked around for help, and a whisper came out of my mouth; "help."

A man was standing at the crossing and he pointed to a barricade and sign that he had placed behind my car. I felt safe. The man yelled; "Ambulance is on the way!"

I relaxed somewhat and looked at the man. I thought that I could see long transparent wings on him. I felt my legs, checked for other injuries. I saw that no fatal injuries were involved and I relaxed thankfully. Then I was shocked to recognize the man's voice; It was Eulogio's voice; The man in the river dreams. I felt as though I was falling through space. When I came to my senses, I was covered with blankets, and two men were carrying me into the hospital.

I was placed in a bed and no one came to see what was wrong for a long time. I was wondering; What is going to happen?" I was sure that I had no serious injuries. Finally, a maid came in and started to clean. I asked her; "Will you do me a favor?" She nodded. I offered her a slip of paper I had and told her; "Please. Call this person and tell her that I am hurt. Ask her to come over."

My friend arrived shortly. She made sure that all the paper work was in good order she checked the insurance records. She made sure that I was going to be fine while she went to the office to provide insurance records. A nurse came soon to clean the glass particles off my skin. She used a brush and a washcloth to scrub the shoulder and arm. Then she disinfected the skin. Later, an Oral Health Provider and his assistant came to see the damage in my mouth.

The Oral Health Provider said to his assistant: "She will need a full bridge."

The Assistant made commiserating sounds that meant to be comforting as she held my hand. There were four teeth missing on the left side of the maxilla where I hit the wheel. Next, a Doctor came to take care of the cuts. The Doctor stitched the loose skin on the nose and lips. The Oral Health Provider and assistant returned to remove small bone splinters from the maxilla. Where the teeth had broken off, tiny splinters were left I was told. It was years later that I remembered these facts. And they were very important. It indicated that there was a plan in the providers' mind.

First; He determined that this was going to be a full bridge. And that was the reason for the partial "not to work out well". A four-teeth partial could have been redone. Instead he planned a full bridge. Therefore, I was misinformed with a purpose.

Second; They returned the same night to remove splinters. Latter on when he sued me, (and I countered.) he denied having removed the splinters himself. But, no other health practitioners or Doctors did any work inside of my mouth until after he sued me.

6

THE PARTIAL BRIDGE

The Man identified as Oral Health Provider waited for the gums to heal and then set up an appointment to start treatment. First; he made a set of four teeth to replace the missing ones. They called it a "temporary." Or a "partial" It was not very helpful with speech, but it was not corrected. The word "temporary," used to describe the partial, made me think that it meant a short time.

After a few weeks, I returned to ask when I was going to get permanent teeth made. I had no idea what all this work meant and the "temporary" was really bad. It made sounds when I spoke.

Air went between the gums and the partial. It did not stay in place.

Finally, I was provided with an appointment to begin working on a full bridge. Now, my trials begin because they did not do the work right. I did not know what to expect. I was not given instructions nor was I informed that my own teeth were going to be cut to hold the bridge which they called the "permanent bridge". There were no forms made to show me the stages of the full bridge that would be done. Neither drawings or photographs. No information to the patient.

I was provided with an appointment to begin working on the full bridge. I was looking forward to it because it would be a relief from discomfort. Instead, difficulties became pain and issues with the bridge. Which turned out to be a "temporary" full bridge before the "final", "permanent"

So, it seems that the patient was led to believe that this bridge would be a permanent item. But they were preparing a "temporary" bridge made of a temporary material.

I did not know at that time that a professional would have made a prototype to use as a model and to show me what the work would be like before cutting my own teeth. I was not even told that my teeth were going to be cut to hold the bridge. NOT A DRAWING OR A SKETCH

At the time, I was going through so many problems that I was really unable to see what was going on. Under normal circumstances, I would have asked for more information than I received. The attitude towards me, made me feel and actually believe that I was the problem; Complaining too much. That problems were my fault. Still, I was patient.

7

CUTTING OF TEETH

On the day of my appointment, there I was sitting on the Dentist's chair with the Practitioner drilling. And the Assistant providing something to help with the pain. It felt like my teeth were being cleaned. I had that work done many times. There was no feeling at all. When I reported feeling "strange" and "I am fainting", The Practitioner stopped the drill and the assistant handed me a mirror to see "the work" done on my teeth.

I looked at my teeth; which had been cut into pointed forms; like Dracula's teeth in cartoon style

I only could murmur; "I didn't know you were doing

this." And repeated in a whisper "I did not Know." As if talking to myself. I could not believe what I was seeing.

The Practitioner looked at his assistant and asked; "Did you show her the forms?

She responded; "I thought that you had…"

This was a sham. They both walked out because they knew that no forms had been made to show their client. They only made molds after the teeth had been cut to a point. The assistant returned and showed me the "temporary bridge." The teeth were not very nice looking. Assistant explained: "You will wear this only until your mouth becomes familiar with it." (Which I suspected it was not true. They had no "final' bridge made yet.") It could not be done without a form. Or so I thought.

I whispered in wonder; "Those teeth are so big." As I considered the looks of the bridge. The assistant went out to consult. Both returned and he explained in a patient tone; "These teeth are the right size for an American woman." He was not having a good day.

I was feeling faint, but I responded with a tinge of irony: "What makes you think that I need that size of teeth? My teeth were half that size, I look like Bugs Bunny." I tried to relax and asked him, "Didn't you see the photograph that you requested for the purpose of looking at my normal looks? And added; "My normal teeth are small."

The assistant reassured me that my permanent teeth were going to be made of porcelain. "This bridge Is made to cover your own teeth until the permanent one is done."

The temporary bridge was made of a material that absorbed food aromas and it stank all the time. Washing it did not help much, nor did any drug store products. Assistant had given me a brush an electric gadget, and all kinds of things to clean my gums. But whenever the bridge came unglued, and I called for an appointment, everyone in the office became unglued too. They had no patience with me anymore. I felt embarrassed and humiliated by this situation; I felt weakened by the pain.

Whenever someone did not recognize me, I tried to be a good sport, but my face had many scars, and these teeth protruding and slanted made my speech strange and difficult to manage. I could see that they had not made allowances for the effect that the removal of bone splinters was now causing. It had been a problem even with the first temporary partial bridge. Whether I spoke in English or Spanish it did not matter, my speech was bad. Whenever I saw my reflection, I felt like another person. I looked terrible and felt even worse. People were very nice to me, but I looked as bad as I felt. I did not recognize myself. This was not me.

I had to return several times because the bridge would become unglued. At the time I did not know, but the bridge was curved incorrectly. So that it came unglued just by chewing. I ate mostly liquids and soft foods. I reported that only one side reached the lower teeth. The other side was not touching. When I spoke, the right side of the bridge hit my lower molar over and over. My jaw hurt most of the time. The bridge curvature was dislocating the jaw. When I mentioned this new pain, the Dentist and the Assistant, both answered; "We have not done any work on your lower teeth. You cannot blame us for that."

The "temporary" full bridge continued to come off over and over. They had to replace it, but the pain continued. The assistant encouraged me by saying that the permanent bridge would be corrected to avoid further problems.

At this point, the pain symptoms had spread to the neck, the ear, the shoulder. I could feel on the side of my neck a nerve that felt like a rope.

8

THE PERMANENT BRIDGE

The final bridge was made exactly like the first. The teeth size seemed to be the same. Besides, the molar on the back hit first when chewing. The bite had not been corrected at all. There was no hope of relief any more.

I reported; "My own jaw teeth are hurting. Porcelain teeth on the new bridge hit like a rock"

I had now porcelain teeth. A stone pounding on the back molar.

They both made the same excuse; "We did not do any work on that tooth. It is not our fault if it hurts."

The bridge became loose often and it was replaced several times. The assistant explained that they were using a temporary glue to make sure that the bridge fitted properly, before installing it permanently.

Finally, patience wore off totally. The assistance decided to install the bridge permanently. Now it would not come off even if they tried.

Apparently, neither the Oral Care Provider nor the Assistant could diagnose the reason for the bridge to come loose. Instead, it was glued on permanently, I certainly reported enough times, and gave a description of the problem. It seems that they did not believe me or did not wish to deal with the mistakes they had made in their work.

The pain continued and finally the molar affected fell off. The bridge now pounded on the next tooth. Amazingly, neither the professional or the Assistant could believe that I was in pain.

One day, as I walked out of consulting with the Oral Care Provider. And I was outraged because the Oral Care Provider Prescribed Nembutal for the pain. (So, he accepted that I was in pain.) I was outraged because the Oral Care Provided prescribed Nembutal, instead of correcting the bridge. This pain had been consistent through out the work on the "partial" and two complete bridges. The only change was that pain increased and spread throughout the area.

When he handed me a prescription, I responded; "YOU! take Nembutal." And walked out to face the Front office attendant handing me a bill. As I looked at the bill, she commented to someone that I must be in love with him and made excuses to see him. (That is what I heard.)

I looked up and responded as softly as I could; "No Mam. I am not IN LOVE. I am IN PAIN. And this office did not do the work right. I want to remind you that I have paid, already, much more than $4,000. 00 and I want my money back."

I went to my car and sat there wondering. Now What? Nembutal gave my head a jolt. It had been prescribed for my aunt. After surgery, she did not heal properly and was given Nembutal for the pain. She became addicted and walked around all night unable to sleep. She finally went to a different Doctor who did surgery again to see what was wrong. A bandage strip had been found inside the wound which had caused an infection. She had been given Nembutal for pain instead of checking what went wrong with the surgery. It also took a long time to recover from addiction.

I knew that pain killers are not a solution. Pain is a symptom that something is wrong. Therefore, I knew that something was very wrong with my teeth, my jaw or both.

I sat in my car wondering what to do next. I felt relieved that I had made a choice. I finally understood that these professionals were abusive. They simply did not know how to do this work. The problem with my teeth, originally, had not been bad enough to cause all this pain and expense. I started the car and felt ready to take charge, I could make choices with confidence. I knew very professional Dentists who could make corrections and do excellent work.

Two days later, I received a notice that my Oral Care

Provider had filed a suit in Court for $1,700. This action confirmed my evaluation of them. "They are actually abusive people." Making mistakes or failing at something can always be resolved. They did not have any intention of making an effort to make amends. Instead they went to court to force me to pay.

I decided to just bite the bullet and take care of myself. This situation was more difficult than ever. Now, I would have to deal with attorneys and expenses that I could not afford. I also had to find a dentist who would be willing to make corrections on the bridge. I was confident because all the Dentists that I knew were capable of doing excellent work.

THE BOARD

I asked the Board to look at this case. Possibly, I could avoid Court Proceedings. My request was accepted. However, The results were incredible. I wanted to avoid court proceedings by having the Board members look into the issue. And this is how it went:

Before the hearing, the Board had assigned two Professional men to evaluate the dental work in my mouth. When we met, One of the Assigned Evaluator said to me. "People with problems like that, usually commit suicide. You will commit suicide."

I considered this statement as we stood outside the office. And I concluded that the Evaluator of Dental work wanted me to commit suicide. That he wanted to implant in my mind that choice. Like the man, the practitioner, who had said to his assistant: "She will need a complete bridge" when I was under the effects of a car crash.

I responded to this Man assigned by the Board; "No, I will not commit suicide, but you are wishing that I do that."

Next: I was provided a hearing where the Committee determined that;

A) Occlusion has been affected by the bridge.

B) Perio Problems.

C) Esthetic problems.

Bridge seems to fit properly.

The first determination: A; means; in plain English, that the bridge caused the jaw to become dislocated, which causes teeth not to meet correctly. And it hurts like hell!

The second problem; B: "perio" periodontal disease which causes gums to bleed.

The Dentist hung a full bridge on sick gums.

And thirdly; C; "Esthetic Problems" meaning: looks like Bugs Bunny, "Bridge SEEMS to fit Properly." The Board Committee ignores the fact that nobody wants to have teeth sticking out, slanted, and hurting.

Not only was the board accepting poor dental work from a member of the profession, but the Professional who accepted to work on my teeth and agreed to be a professional witness in Court, if needed, was threatened by his peers, members of the same profession.

We had started to work on removing the bridge that had been attached PERMANENTLY, and it was the most difficult experience for me and for the professional. Besides living with the twisted bridge for months.

This professional was threatened by other peers from the community. Many who had turned me down when I asked for corrections. We discussed the issue. And determined that he could not provide expert witness evidence in court. We did not know how far these people were willing to go.

I agreed readily and accepted. I said to him 'I know what kind of people we are dealing with. I agree that you will not testify in court. You take care of your family.

This good Man corrected the bridge and it lasted for several months before the joint started to change, as he had predicted. This kind of damage stays for life. And yes, some people commit suicide to avoid suffering. This dentist made corrections and soon after, he closed his office. He moved away from town.

As soon as I chose another practitioner to make corrections. He received threats. He was told that he would not be allowed to be a witness in court and he would not be able to purchase materials needed to do his work

Here again, we have professionals threatened. The two professional highly respected health providers are threatened. This is done to protect one man who did a horrible job and then sued his client.

The evaluations made actually reported that the

chances of recovery from this kind of damage to my jaw were: NO CHANCE!

Actually, the corrections made would change. It continued to change and to cause pain just as all the dentists that I consulted with had told me. I considered my options and decided that I needed to remove the bridge and and remove the teeth that had been cut to hold the bridge. Of course, everyone said that it was madness. And I agreed. "Yes, this is madness, but that is the best I can do now" Most people have experienced tooth ache sometime in life. It is horrible! Nobody wants to face a lifetime of being exposed to this kind of pain at any time, for life.

My decision came from research that I had been doing. I spent time in the San Diego Medical Library where I discovered that it was practically impossible to correct this work effectively, because it does change. The work itself is painful and expensive. VERY expensive. However; "Curanderos" are able to treat bones and joints with some effectiveness. And it is done without pain and in a short time. I found this out during the same search.

In a particularly bad day that I was having. My brother picked me up and took me to the "curandero" and the man did return the jaw back, with one motion. It stayed in place for months.

Needless to say. I make it a habit to never disclose who or what practitioner of what medicine provides treatment to me. Just to avoid threats or distress for providing health care to me.

Neither do I disclose any health providers' names to avoid distress of other people involved in the system.

This kind of damage usually happens with a blow to the jaw or car accidents. That is why the first Practitioner and his assistant felt that he could blame the problem on his client's automobile accident. And ignore reports of pain. Only that he did not expect his client to do research. Besides there were two written reports of professionals, testifying for the Court that dental work caused the damage.

THE BREAKDOWN

There is a good reason for a breakdown. You can only go up from there:

Meantime, I was making efforts to get a job I took a summer class that was required for teachers. I was feeling rather weak and tired, but the University and change of airs helped. However, I was not so strong. I had a breakdown during class. One day the teacher asked that we write down one issue that we needed to work on. I started to write. And about two lines down I put my pencil on the desk, picked up my purse and walked out. I went home, got in bed and stayed there.

About three days later a friend noticed that I was not going to classes and went to check on me. When she knocked on the door, I got up and let her in. She could see immediately that I was not well. She asked me if I had any objections to seeing a psychiatrist. I said "no" with my head. She took me to one she knew, and waited for me. Then she fed me, took me home, and put me in bed to rest.

I have no memory of what was said or done. Except that on the last day, I was ready to go home. My psychiatrist, recommended a book for me to follow and do exercises. He felt that I was well enough to do it on my own. The book provided me with information and exercises to do. It also led to other self help books and recordings. I learned to relax, to change my beliefs, to stop pain. After a while, I made my own recordings to focus on my needs. The problems don't just go away, but it helps to develop skills to overcome pain. I made improvements, even though the problems have lasted all my life.

I had once a rather spiritual experience;

I woke up one day and the pain was totally out of hand. I could not open a can to eat. Everything hurt.

I thought "Even my hair hurts." I walked out of the house, automatically, practically dragged my feet and took my body to a bench behind the house. Just sat there, not thinking. Then I started to slide off the bench and sat on the ground. I felt the need to lower my head (Like someone was pushing my head down) I touched the ground with my forehead and I felt relief. The pain just faded away. And I experienced peace. After a few minutes, I started to notice my position. I thought; "My position is like that of Muslims when they pray to God." Then wondered; "Is my head pointing towards Mecca?" And next; I realized that: "I do not know where I am or where the city of Mecca is." Then I considered "It is fine, I guess. We pray to the same God."

I experienced a deep sense of relief, peace, strength. I made up my mind to take that position whenever I felt pain from the jaw. And, of course, Thanked God for this experience.

Sidney Petrie in association with Robert B. Stone PhD. Helping Yourself with Autogenetics.

11

THE DEVIL'S ADVOCATE

A LOCAL ATTORNEY ADVISED ME THAT I NEEDED A SPECIALIST; A MALPRACTICE ATTORNEY.

There was only one Malpractice Attorney in the big city, nearby. This meant trips from the farm to the city, and /or phone calls. The attorney wasted time in many ways. First; he decided to wait and see what the Board of Dental Examiners would decide. In time, he had me respond to questions. The Dentist left town and responded to his questions months later. My attorney told me that there was nothing to do but wait for him to return. In other words; "When hell frizzes over."

That is what I understood. He also gave me a choice. "You are free to get another attorney or represent yourself. I will not be offended." I listened quietly and told myself; "Good Malpractice Attorneys don't grow on trees."

Letters were not acknowledged, trips to speak to him did not help. He became offended that I was not patient. He had not even filed a Counterclaim in Court. Then I wondered if I was wrong in thinking that he was my attorney because we did not have a contract on file.

Months and years had passed. One day, I drove to the big City to clarify what he had done so far He gave me then the "Devil's advocate" bit about what could happen. And he then repeated that If I did not like his work, I could represent myself.

My time had been spent in looking up any legal information that could help me. Then I found that I had access to the Law Library. There also a summer program for Legal Assistants in San Diego. I signed up to learn about process, paper work, legal forms etc.

The last appointment with my attorney had been very polite and agreeable, words were the same. I knew he was not going to do anything for me. He said once more "If you do not like my work, you can represent yourself. You are a good speaker and very able person."

I listened quietly. He saw me as such a stupid person. He did not think that I could understand what he was doing. He actually acted as though there was really no choice for me. I stood up slowly and said quietly; "Please, Sir. Will you remove yourself from the case?"

He looked surprised, and I started to walk away to leave. At the door, I turned around and said to him; "You know something? A woman like me; sick, stupid, ignorant! Can do a better job than you any day." I walked out and stood outside. Listening.

He recovered from his surprise and started yelling at his secretary; Angry, loud, orders. I knew the signs now. I took a deep breath and told myself; "Yep! He does not want to do this work, but he expects me to wait indefinitely."

During my drive home, I wondered about myself. How is it that I am falling at the hands of people like that? This is no accident; that my oral Health Provider, the board, my Attorney are all neglecting their work and obligations. I placed my trust on them and they failed to perform. I acknowledged that I had made these poor choices, but now I needed to take care of my needs.

Pain and distress are the reasons I had for fighting my way through. But I must watch my choices.

My life had never been like that. No one ever treated me so badly.

At some instances, I considered that the attorney was right to take care of his business. I am not a client that will return for further services. The professionals; businesses, industry are important clients for an attorney. However, he accepted me to represent in court and just keeps me dangling without performing meaningful work. We had no contract at all. That was a bad sign for me. And my health deteriorated further with all this stress.

12

PREPARATION TO
ANSWER "THE CALL"

When the summer came, I went to San Diego for Paralegal Classes. Three moths of research and intensive work. I became acquainted with other students and mainly two women. One introduced herself as a witch; "Anyone who needs my services, please ask." The other lady was very wise. I called her the Wise Goddess." We did work together and went out to find books and goodies that San Diego had to offer. When I refused to go out because I was working on my legal papers, they wanted to know about it. The Wise goddess became concerned that I would not be able to reach my goal. She tried to dissuade me from it. Finally, she said to me. "O.K. girl! This is my pearl of wisdom to you. Pay close attention to what the Judge says." I did pay attention and did as I was told. The judge's every word was an important part of the process for me.

The Witch was also interested in my project. She offered that I accept her craft and use her craft for help. I considered it and decided; "No, I want to make all the choices by myself."

I did progress and I was offered a chance to continue in the University to become an attorney, but I did not think that I would fit in.

My next step was to write a request for the Court to remove my Attorney: Kitchen/Office combination. I made purchases that were needed. A Xerox copier, an electric typewriter; a Brother. Paper, Law Dictionary and so on. I was ready for the next step. Usually, I over prepare for any thing that I want to do. I wanted to make the Judge's work easy to do. Therefore; I over prepared.

I did most of my research and made copies of forms,

and so on in San Diego. Everything went well. I started to believe that I was now receiving protection from above. Some serious protection. But, of course, I was working day and night practically. There were many times when I faced something that was difficult to do. And the answer would appear right in front of me.

One day I was enjoying a moment where I had accomplished a difficult finding in law. My nephew came in just as I was laughing and shaking my fists in the air, and I did a little dance.

My nephew said; "What are you doing? You witch! A law dance?" Implying that I was doing a "rain dance". He joined in and declared. "Those guys don't know what they are in for. Do they?"

13

RETURNING TO TOWN, MANY PEOPLE SHOWED CONCERN

People in town had started to notice what I was doing and there was great distress from people who felt that I was causing harm to the Oral Health Practitioner. At this point, the man returned to town because he knew I had no attorney and I was representing myself. There were two instances when a person showed special interest in the case.

One male teacher who saw me enter a Pizza place and he called me over. I thought: "What is this? He has never acknowledged that I exist. And now he knows my name?

So he spoke to me: "What is this I hear? You are suing your Dentist? Don't you know that he is going to lose everything he has worked for? He has worked very hard to achieve his position."

He stopped and looked at me fixedly while his wife did the same. She agreed with the question and then put in her two cents. The teacher spoke to me as he would speak to his cook, or his maid, or a child. I did not like that. Even if I had been a maid.

Then I answered; "You are misinformed. The man took me to court because I refused to pay for his bad work. I have paid already around $5,000. And he is making me look like I don't pay my bills. He is abusing his position."

I felt that this was a chance to let "others" know why I was in court, and explained further: "He made me a bad bridge that is crooked and it dislocated my jaw joint. He also cut my teeth to place his crooked bridge on them. This bridge makes my joint come out whenever it is attached in place again. This Dentist made the same mistake three times; First he made a partial that was bad. Then he made a temporary bridge with the same faults, and finally he made a permanent bridge with the same faults. Not only that but his assistant used permanent glue or something that forced me to suffer having it removed. A very painful job. This means that he did not want to make corrections or he did not know how to make them."

I took a breath and noticed that I had just gone on too long. They looked shocked and I just went on encouraged; "This "Professional" is taking the legal system to blame his client and make me look like a low down sort of person; Which, as you might know is against the law AND WHICH YOU might also know is that the first thing an abusive person does is DISCREDIT THE VICTIM." The last thing I wanted to say came faster: "Most importantly, any compensation that I might receive is never going to change the damages that he caused. I have to live with it" Then, I smiled a big "Polite" smile towards each one and said; "thank you for asking."

Both looked surprised and confused. They had been misinformed. Both stuttered and stared at each other with a look of incredulity. I walked away to join my friend.

The second person was a woman.

An unknown woman approached me. She said that she had been looking for me and asked my name. She wanted to tell me that I should work to the end in the matter. "That man!" She said and became emotional. She continued speaking faster; She explained that the professional provided dental care to children who were under Government custody; "He does bad work and the children cry in pain." The children are taken regularly for dental care, and soon they are crying in pain. She said: "The response is always; They just want attention."

The woman reported that it happened to many children. She wanted to prevent him from doing dental work. "Children don't cry for attention all night" She said sternly. The woman appeared outraged and helpless. She had to take the children to him because there was a contract or something that made it an obligation for her to take the children to him.

I reassured her that I had no intention of letting it go. I agreed with her. This man should not be practicing in that profession I told her that her request made me even more determined to prevent other people from being harmed through poor dental work.

14

THE LEGAL WORK CONTINUES

I typed my papers carefully and even started again if a sentence was broken in the middle I wanted it to be perfect and clear even if it took me a long. Time. Whenever I had a doubt, I went to the local legal library where I could read cases, statutes, copy forms, I started to feel terrified and at the same time, excited. I felt better when one of my friends offered to go with me on the Court date. I accepted happily; "Yes, I am afraid that I might need someone to pick me up if I faint."

When we arrived to the building, I noticed that my Attorney was driving a Mercedes and his brother, also an Attorney, was with him. That gave me a wave of relief and said to my Friend; "So, I am not the only one who needs support."

I had lots of papers with me. I had noticed that papers I filed in court were not on file. Surely, The Opposition was removing them. I had seen him go in every time I was there. So I made sure to have extra copies of my records: my Counterclaim, and a request to remove my Legal Representative on File. I wanted to hand the copies to the Judge personally. Not taking any chances!

The Local Representative had requested an informal setting for the hearing. And the Opposition had changed it to a formal setting. It did not matter to me, but it was one more sample of his "style". Must be a tough style to live.

15

THE COURT HEARING

When the Honorable Judge Plath walked in, I handed him a copy of my work. After customary proceedings, he took a look at my papers and gave me a quick look. Asking; "Who helped you to do the legal paper work?"

I responded; "I did the work myself Sir."

The Honorable Judge Plath explained as he looked at the work; "Someone had to help you or someone did it for you. This is very well done."

I smiled and repeated; "I did the work myself, Sir. I do research.".

H. Judge Plath made doubtful sounds and waved his hands over the papers insisting; "This is; not only research. Someone did this work for you and he or she will get in trouble for it. "Maybe a two-year Law student?" He continues reading some parts.

He shakes his head in denial. "Can't be."

I explained; "Yes, I have been working on this for about two years. I started to do dental research first because I am in pain. Then I started to do legal research in the Law Library. Besides, I took classes at the University of San Diego. It has taken lots of time and work.

I stopped and took a deep breath. I looked at the Honorable Judge Plath directly, feeling fearful and somewhat stupid.

H. Judge Plath patiently explains. "It does not matter what you have learned. This work is very well done. I wish attorneys would be as careful and specific as this one is. I cannot believe that you did this work."

Later, I thought that he said that for the benefit of the attorneys; there was no work from them on file. I also know that because, I received my Attorney's file after he was removed from the case and he had been paid. There were only letters from one attorney to the other, back and forth describing what document should be written and filed. Just notes for which he was paid top dollar. Not legal process documents. He did not even have a Contract with me.

I smiled at the Honorable Judge Plath words and responded; "Thank you Sir. Your words sound like I get an "A" for my work I am very glad that it is acceptable legal work."

Things got a little sticky, I could see that the problem was serious for Judge Plath

How could he accept this documentation? And how could he leave a woman without legal representation?

Actually, that was the main Issue. I asked for my Legal Representative to be removed from the case. And I blurted out without thinking; "Why can't it be accepted that I did this work? Is it because I am a woman? or because I am from another culture?"

The H. Judge Plath laughed and said "I better accept it or you will end up suing me."

I said respectfully; "No Sir. I would not sue you!"

And I thought; "I also know that I would be is serious legal trouble (jail even) if I misrepresent to the Court"

H. Judge Plath then directed his questions to the attorneys; My Attorney, his brother, who is an Attorney also, the local Attorney assisting in the case, and the Oral Care Practitioner's Attorney.

My Representative asked that he be paid for his work if I received any money. (What gall. I have to negotiate and do the work, but he wants to get paid. He always told me that the case was not "worth much" anyway. But, I was willing to pay to get him off the case.

The Local Representative agreed to stay on the case. And I agreed too.

There were other questions and money responsibilities.

I insisted; I do not see why my Representative never got me an appointment to speak to the Insurance. Then

I asked; Isn't that the first step? I am waiting for years to get out of court. Being sued in court is shameful for me because I never fail to pay my debts. The Insurance will not speak to me. They speak only to the Legal Representative. And he tells me that my problem is not serious, that I will get some miserly sum of money.

There was an attempt to have Legal Representation and me agree to something. But everyone got a chance to observe how rude he acted towards me. And he was being more patient than usual. Besides, I did not want to continue dealing with him. I could not agree to anything after all that time wasted waiting for him to work on this case.

I listened carefully to what H. Judge Plath said. The Insurance would be informed that the attorney is off the case and to speak to me. I made an appointment right away and soon went to meet with the insurance.

The Honorable (Fictitious name due to privacy rights) Cause ----------

19----- Superior Court

16

THE PRACTITIONER'S INSURANCE

I made an appointment with the insurance and drove to the Big City for the meeting. There was no trouble. At first I was told that only attorneys could speak to them. I told the Receptionist that the Attorney had been removed from the case, and that I was representing myself. It seems that they already knew about it and I was given an appointment.

I had everything in order and my argument was on a list. A long list. One of the main arguments was actually a statement. "Your Insured changed the Medical Records to show that I had suffered TMJ in the accident."

She looked at me disdainfully; "And what do I care about that? What does it matter to me?

I explained; "He lied for to reasons; First; He wanted to make it look like I suffered TMJ in the accident when he actually caused the damage. Second: My insurance would have paid much more if I had a dislocated jaw than four teeth lost in the accident.

Tough Woman replied; "And so what?" (not a question but a bark!)

My smile turns into a bitter laugh; "Your boss might want to know that your insured is committing insurance fraud."

I continued: This professional wants a client with lots of money. It has cost me already around $6,000 for one bridge that causes me pain. The Dentist expected that he would make several bridges and never be right again. Lots of expensive work to be provided.

I took several pieces of dental work to show how crooked they were. And placed them on the table. Tough

Woman made a wry face and said; "UGH! TAKE THAT OUT OF MY SIGHT!"

"Tough Woman" started to walk to the exit; I spoke louder; "Your client wants me to wear it." "Tough Woman" stopped at the door and said; "I will offer you $50:000 NO MORE! And I answered: "NO THANKS!" BEFORE THE DOOR SLAMMED SHUT,

I had to consider that the offer was nothing compared to the expenses that I would have in the future. Just getting a new bridge would be around $6,000. each time. And I still did not know what other effects I would experience as a result of the faulty bridge. Other damages were coming up. And my health in general suffered the effects of pain.

I picked up my things and said "Thank you" to the gentlemen sitting at the table. I thought: "hopefully they are investors.". No one had been introduced nor did "Tough Woman" introduced herself. It seems that the quality of insurance personnel declines as they climb the success ladder.

17

THE INSURANCE ATTORNEY PLAYS THE LAST CARD

The Tantalizing offer:

The insurance continues to make offers; I received a written offer by mail where the offer is a much larger sum than the one made by "Tough Woman". But the conditions were that it would be provided on a monthly basis. The writer is trying to entice me by insinuating that the offer is "Tantalizing". I responded; "It is interesting that you should call this offer "Tantalizing".

As far as I know it means that you get it but you don't Is this too profound for you?

Well, it is like this; Tantalos was sent to hell where he would suffer the well known hot conditions.

He was a son of Zeus, He was sent to hell because of his "Hubris" (Pride; He offended the Gods of Olympus) Well he could never get water or food. He was placed in a pool of water with a fruit tree right above him. The water and fruit came to his mouth and withdrew when he opened his mouth to drink or eat.

As you can see; the fact that you are using this word. Tells me what you are thinking, or the insurance is thinking. Your choice of words tells me that you and the insurance are playing games.

Besides, I can handle my own money just fine, I don't need someone to handle it.

So, Get serious,

Then, I Wrote; "Tantalizing means that you do not get it. Clear and simple. It does not mean tempting. That is what I responded; MORE OR LESS.

SOON AFTER, I received a notice that a hearing

would be held and that my Health Provider was filing bankruptcy. I went to the hearing and the Office Manager, was present. I thought, "Yep! She does all the management work,"

He is supposed to be taking some classes. But he reappeared as soon as he heard that I was representing myself. He still had hopes.

18

MY HEALTH PROVIDER SUING ME DECLARES BANKRUPTCY

I received a letter from one of the Attorneys. It informed me that the man who was suing me would be filing bankruptcy. (So he was not going to pay the professional who sold him the practice.) The man who sued me for payment, will not pay his debt. I wonder, what does this tell me about the man? He uses the legal process for everything.

The young Attorney called me as soon as he received his notice. He seemed to enjoy his position. He said; "This is over. That's it! The suit is over!"

And continued; "You should have taken the offer

of settlement. You will not get anything now because bankruptcy means that he does not have to pay his debts."

He stops for a moment and I respond; "Sounds like him to do this."

The young Attorney was young and proud of himself. He is having fun with it. And he repeats; "Like ...it's over! We are winning!" (He's happy, full of joy, not really mean.)

I say to him: "let me check it out, and I will answer soon."

Since this was fun, he could not resist repeating; "This is it! There is no more!"

I insisted: "I will respond by mail, soon!"

I headed for the Law Library, and was able to see what he was filing under, Not hard! It was on the Notice. I read the conditions, made notes and went home to write a response for the young attorney. The response informed the attorney that his client was not going to pay me, therefore, His debt to me will not be cancelled. And I sent it.

As soon as he received it he called me again. He was surprised, He insisted: "bla, bla. bla talking very fast; "This is BANKRUPTCY! Do you know what that means?"

I responded: "His insurance will pay once we agree on an amount," His surprise was even greater. He did not try to hide it. "I cannot believe my ears." He mumbled "How did you find out so fast?" He continued under his breath; "I know that you received the Notice late yesterday, And I have your response already,"

I answered: "Well? First I checked the law that he is filing under. Then I wrote an answer to mail it by overnight mail. You seemed to be anxious to receive an answer?" This was sort of a question.

He insisted; "That is incredible! An attorney would have taken two months, or so, to research an answer."

My answer was ironical; "I know that, but I am not an attorney" Too bad, irony was lost on him.

The gentleman really wanted to know HOW! "How do you do it? Someone has to be telling you what to do." He was speaking in earnest.

I responded nicely; "Thank you, I will take that as a compliment. I have worked very hard in this matter because my attorney would not do it."

He stutters; "But how can you DO! it?

I respond; each word separately; in a low tone; "I-give-a-dammed-hot."

I should have said; "because I care" but it came out of my deepest pain-filled insides with intensity. He was very quiet for a moment. And then we parted.

19

SETTLEMENT

I agreed to a settlement because I wanted to be out of court and continue my life away from dangerous people. I did not want to expose other professionals, who helped me to make corrections in my mouth, to be dragged into a court as reluctant witnesses. The threats they received were real.

"Professionals?" I wonder how many children went through the abuse and pain I suffered?" But the Honorable Judge Plath accepted my work and DID THE RIGHT THING.

At the end, a team of attorneys was representing the Oral Health Practitioner. They needed a team of man to trick the stupid old woman showing their disrespect over and over. It seems that it never entered their mind "DO THE RIGHT THING"

As for myself, I believe that I was meant to go through these higher levels of pain-filled experience so that I might grow in wisdom. I have forgiven those people for their transgressions against me. Their transgressions against children is something that I cannot believe. I believe that there has been no change in the health professions. People who are abusive WILL abuse the system.

Publishing this experience, provides readers with information that is needed when having work done in any part of the body, or any kind of health services.

Having to trust health practitioners or trust unknown health providers is always a risk. The competence level accepted by the professionals is a crime. And the RESPONSIBILITY level shown by those that I met within the profession is unspeakable. And I do not mean those professionals who do their best. It is a difficult life and there are many good people within the profession.

However, when a committee or a Board accepts that destruction of a person's physical body is acceptable. We need to look again. The Board accepted that the damage to the mouth, jaw, teeth is acceptable because "It can be corrected." That is a high class crime. Not only is it costly in money standards, but The two Oral Health Practitioners that The Board assigned to check the work. Said to me that people commit suicide when they suffer this kind of pain. In fact, it is happening!

I believe that when a health practitioner causes TMJ in a person's mouth he/she ought to pay dearly for it. Not hide behind insurance. They will stop taking one class and advertise that they can make corrections to TMJ. I spent one whole day calling around town anyone who advertised ability to make corrections on TMJ after they took a class in a theatre.

I was able to receive assistance from many people; the good old "wives' tales". A person can find legal information for free in the library. We did not even have computers when I did my research.

In a library. I also found information about "curanderos". "Don Gabino" was respected for his ability to return bones to their proper position. He learned from his ancestors. Not at a university. His "License" was the numerous crutches that hung on his tree. Which were left there when a person did not need it anymore.

My Grandmother used herbs to cure the community ills. Before medicine came to town. Unfortunately, for me she was already dead when I needed it. I had to discover it by myself.

Modern Medicine has made great advances and practitioners are really good. How unfortunate that it fails sometimes.

My experience led me to function at a higher level. I have learned and worked on things that never would have been part of my life. It has been useful for me. I have grown to know myself and developed great respect for my body, mind, and spirit.

20

IN CLOSING

The dreams about the Colorado River are part of my experience. I did not want to go on the adventure. I have come to the conclusion that my path CAME FOR ME TO TAKE ME THROUGH THE EXPERIENCE. My life was just right before the experience and also after the adventure.

I ask myself' WHAT IS LIFE? There is good and evil. We cannot be all good or all evil.

WE SEARCH FOR THE PLACE THAT IS JUST RIGHT. THE MIDDLE GROUND! THAT IS JUST RIGHT!

The book actually started when I kept a journal of my dreams. (The dreams that happen during sleep. Not the dreams that are WISHES.) And later when I started to journal events that happened during dental work. And with the legal representation. It just did not seem right to me. I did not rely on my memory. Many things happened that were not recorded. A lot of my friends were on the look out for what was going on with the case. Many felt terrible about it because they did not believe that I could represent myself.

Everyone helped as well as they could but the battle felt lonely. The court hearing was the most important point. When The Honorable Judge Plath said 'It does not matter what you have learned. This work is very well done. I wish attorneys would be as careful and as specific as this one is. I cannot believe that you did this work.' He was telling the legal Professionals how they failed to represent their client.

Writing down events in a journal kept my mind clear because I knew that information was available. I did not have to remember it all or fear that my mind would fail me.

I hope that many people will notice how important dental work is and how devastating its effect when it is done wrong. Even removing an infected tooth can lead to great losses. And an experience of high intensity tooth pain or damaged bone structure is bad enough to affect a child's normal development.

Respectfully;

Dolores Sefirot

About the Author

Readers would benefit from some of the steps taken by author; Dolores Sefirot.

Due to health problems caused by poor dental work, she researched for ways to recover. All kinds of pain treatment were useless. She suffered a breakdown that led to psychiatric care; learning how to overcome pain, stress, loss of normal speech. Eventually she decided that pulling the teeth that held the bridge, would help. It did help.

Legal services failed too. This led to legal research. She represented herself answering to the Dentist who sued her for fees she refused to pay. At 50 years-old she went to study again; Masters in Education with Emphasis in Psychology and worked as a Licensed Professional Counselor. She retired at 72 years-old.

Dolores wants readers to see how a problem that seemed impossible to resolve was overcome with the help of all the Dentists, Psychiatrist, Writers, Court that provided their skills to overcome similar situations.